Taiji Notebook
for Martial Artists

Essays by a
Yang Family Taijiquan
Practitioner

by Scott M. Rodell

Seven Stars Books and Video

Annandale, Virginia

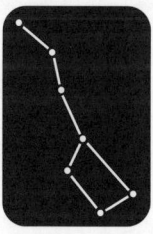

www.sevenstarstrading.com

Published by Seven Stars Books and Video

copyright: Scott M. Rodell 1991

Printed in the United States of America

No part of this book may be used or reproduced in any manner whatsoever without the written permission of the author except in the case of brief quotations embodied in critical articles and reviews.

Cover calligraphy by Chen Dadong

Library of Congress Control Number: 2005903426
isbn: 0-9743999-3-0

For information:
Seven Stars Trading Co., 3543 Marvin Street, Annandale, VA 22003-1712
www.sevenstarstrading.com

All Rights Reserved

Acknowledgements

I would like to thank the many teachers and classmates who help me in my study of *taijiquan*. I am particularly indebted to my principle teacher, Wang Yen-nien, T.T. Liang -- though he is no longer with us, he will never be forgotten -- and WIlliam C. C. Chen for their instruction.

I would also like to thank those who gave so many hours to reading, editing and proofing this book: Bede Bidlack, Seth Davis, Clinton C. Rodell, Steve M. Roth, Jonathan Rollins, Greg Wolfson and Doug Mullane. Their suggestions were most helpful.

I also have to thank my sweet wife Meilu. Without her support, I would achieve little in this life...

Disclaimer: Only you are responsible for yourself and for those with whom you train. Neither the author nor the publisher is accountable for your actions. If you hurt yourself or others by practicing anything you read in this book, you are to blame and must accept the responsibility. THE PRACTICE OF *TAIJIQUAN'S* TWO PERSON WORK, LIKE ANY OTHER MARTIAL ART, IS ITSELF A DANGEROUS ACTIVITY. You can absolutely expect to be injured, perhaps seriously, in the course of study and practice. That is the nature of serious training in any martial art, this one included. Go forward with your head up and your eyes open.

A Note on Spelling-

I have chosen to use the newer pinyin spelling, replacing the better known, old Wade-Giles transliteration of Mandarin. For example, *t'ai chi ch'uan* (often misspelled and shortened to tai chi) is spelled *taijiquan* in this text. The only exception to this is for proper names, in which case I have used that person's own spelling of his or her name to avoid confusion. In the case of historical figures, I have generally used the pinyin spelling with the older Wade-Giles in parentheses the first time the name appears in the text. One notable exception to this is for the well-known teacher, Cheng Man-ch'ing, whose name is spelled Zheng Manqing in pinyin. Cheng and this spelling of his name are so well known in America and Europe that updating the spelling of his name would most likely only confuse readers. I know many people still prefer the older spellings to the new pinyin from Mainland China. I was also that way, until a friend reminded me of two important points: the world has changed to pinyin as the internationally accepted spelling of Mandarin in all languages, and it would not do for a Daoist practitioner of *taijiquan* not to be able to change.

Taiji Notebook -
Essays by a Yang Family *Taijiquan* Practitioner

Contents:

Author's Introduction	*xi*
One Question	1
New Students	3
Approaching *Taijiquan*	5
The System	13
The System within the System	19
Slow	21
Flow	25
Fang Song	27
Breathing and *Fajin*	33
Basics	37
Duifang	39
Tuishou - Ting Jin, Dong Jin, and Hua Jin	41
Sanshou	45
Conflict	51
Good and Bad Techniques	53
Technique	57
Supermen and Common People	61
Alert, Inside and Out	65
Mistakes	67
Injury	69
Tournament Competition	71
Fear	75
Opponents	77
Selected Readings	79

Author's Introduction

The words offered here are not the words of a master. They are my thoughts and experiences related to my journey towards mastery. One might well ask what value is there in studying the words of those who have yet to reach the pinnacle of their art? Indeed, I have asked this question of other works, both spoken and written. I also asked this question of myself many times before I decided to write down what I have been teaching my students.

I finally decided to record my experiences for two reasons. The first is that, unfortunately, *taijiquan* is declining as an art both here and in China. The reasons for this are misconceptions among practitioners as to the nature of the art, its most basic concepts, and its methods for the step-by-step development of skills in its practitioners.

The second reason for taking up the pen is that I have learned a great deal from my classmates as well as from my teachers. I have learned from listening to their thoughts and insights. I made progress by watching to see what errors they made so that I might avoid them and shorten my road to mastery. Many practitioners miss this opportunity for learning due to stubbornness. I understand the desire to receive all the teaching directly from one's teacher, but it is foolish to isolate ourselves from every other learning experience. Such isolation can also be a form of arrogance when we think that only we can correctly absorb what the teacher presents and what our classmates have gained is incorrect. I take my differences of opinion with my classmates not as a signal that I am right or wrong but as a sign that none of us has yet fully absorbed the teachings of this art.

Therefore, I have recorded these thoughts as an offering to all students of *taijiquan* following the path to mastery. I sincerely hope you find these words useful and will excuse my errors.

Some of the treatises presented here were written after a particularly strong practice or after reading an enlightening verse. At these times, personal illumination followed the action of training. I reached for the pen and wielded it as a sword, not stopping to examine the last cut but flowing to the next. Some of these treatises may not be as logically organized as others. However, I have only minimally edited these sword/pen works to preserve the feeling of the moment.

What I have written here applies equally to men and women. I firmly believe that a woman can easily equal or better a man if she reaches for the heart of *taijiquan*. Chinese martial his-

Author's Introduction

tory is replete with tales of women who were superior warriors who not only prevailed over many opponents in lethal combat but led armies to victory. In my own experience, women learn and absorb *taijiquan* more quickly than men. Women soften up, relax, and yield more readily than men. Therefore, I have used he/she and have de-gendered my sentences wherever possible. If at any time I wrote "he" alone, it was not meant to exclude women; it was a matter of awkwardness. In these instances, I could just as easily have used "she."

"*Gongfu* (skill) has no end, practice yourself; sharp skill comes from hard work and diligence."
-signed, Yang Zhendou, presented to the author after a training in Taiyuan, China.

Throughout this work, I have chosen to use Chinese terms in place of the English equivalents. I made this choice not because *taijiquan* is exclusively Chinese but because the terminology is. Most of the important, basic concepts and terms do not even have a close equivalent in our language. I feel it is much easier and more meaningful to learn a few new words than to use substitutes, especially when the connotations of these substitutes may only create confusion.

One Question

Occasionally, when a new group of students would join an intermediate-level class, Robert W. Smith* would ask them: "If the greatest master of *taijiquan* were resurrected and stood here, and you could ask him one question, what would you ask?" Everyone searched for the perfect question, including me. No one could ever think of what to ask. Smith instructed us that there was but one question worth asking: "What time is practice?"

---

*I began my study of *Taijiquan* with Smith in Bethesda, Maryland, back in 1980 while I was still at the University. He is well known for the many books he authored on Chinese martial arts and as Cheng Man-ch'ing's first non-Chinese student.

2

New Students

New students signing up for *taijiquan* class do not really expect much. The typical beginner's goal (in America) is "stress relief" and a little exercise. That is not really much to ask of an art that has evolved for hundreds of years.

The real irony of this is that students who seek *taijiquan* instead of heading for the spandex world of franchise gyms want a more "holistic" exercise. That is, they want a system of exercise that addresses the mind and spirit and not just the body. Yet the first thing they do is break the art up into pieces with the statement, "I just want to relax and get a workout. I'm not interested in self-defense or fighting." The way this truly holistic art is designed, there is no separating a proper, dynamic practice that strengthens and loosens the body; improves health and stamina; is a deep form of concentration mediation; and, at the same time, develops clear, practical, martial skills. Everything is connected.

Sometimes when prospective students call

my Center,* I am asked, "Do you teach health *taijiquan* or martial *taijiquan*?" There is only one type of *taijiquan*. The same aspects of training that provide for a strong, healthy body and provide for deep mediation are the tools for learning the martial applications of yielding, neutralizing, and striking.

Instead of foolishly trying to section off and limit our art and practice, we should embrace everything within the art, get everything that we pay for through our practice, and apply it to making life better.

"Martial artist" is not a dirty phrase. Stop and consider the attributes of a good martial artist. First, he or she must be healthy. Without good health, you cannot do much. Second, he needs to be physically fit, something everyone wants to enjoy. And last, a good martial artist has learned how to remain calm. He/she has learned how to stay calm, not just in everyday situations but in uncomfortable, dangerous, and even violent circumstances. In the world we all live in, gaining this last virtue is something that can be useful every day. Even if a student never needs to use *taijiquan* for self-defense, a martial practice is useful every day, for the everyday.

---

*I teach and study *taijiquan* and Chinese Historical Swordsmanship at Great River Taoist Center, headquartered in Washington, D.C., with affiliates and branches in other U.S. cities and in Europe.

Approaching *Taijiquan*

Today, there are millions of people practicing *taijiquan*. In fact, it is likely the most popular form of exercise in the world. This in itself is singularly amazing when we consider that a little over a hundred years ago it was a well-guarded secret of one family in the mountains of Henan province.

Yet *taijiquan* is dying. It's not dying in the sense that it will disappear. Obviously, with people practicing the world over, it is not about to disappear. The art is dying because masters are fewer and fewer in number. And many *taijiquan* experts and living masters feel the time of the great masters may have passed.

How can this be? Does it really make sense? If only one practitioner in 10,000 reaches mastery, with one million people in training we should have 10,000 masters among us. If one in 100,000 achieves this level, we should still have 1,000. And that is assuming there are only one million total practitioners, whereas there are several million *taijiquan* adherents in the world. As the number of masters continues to decline, something is clearly amiss.

The reasons for the art's decline have to do with the approach that contemporary practitioners take to *taijiquan*. In both China and the United States, nearly all take up the art as a health tonic. In Taiwan, the more traditional of the two Chinas, I was regularly laughed at by Chinese of all ages and walks of life -- not for studying *taijiquan* but for studying it now while I am still fairly young, and for beginning while I was in college! To them, *taijiquan* is something old people do in the park.

Approaching *taijiquan* as nothing more than an exercise is precisely what has robbed the art and, more importantly, the practitioners of its value. I do not simply mean the art's martial value but specifically its health and meditative quality.

The reason for this is pure and simple. *Taijiquan* is an internal martial art. It was created out of China's vast martial tradition as a means of deadly defense. This art developed in a society where law extended just a few feet past the city gate; after that, you were on your own. China is, and has been, a culture steeped in the martial tradition (though in ways very different than the more familiar martial tradition of Japan). Every Chinese child knows the story of heroes such as Mulan and Huang Feihong. These heroes are widely respected for their virtue.

The meditative and health aspects of *taijiquan* - this dynamic martial art - are essentially side effects. As valuable and useful as they are, they remain nothing more than this. In order to gain the twin benefits of health and meditation, bodily precision, full spirit, and strong mind intent are required. It is not possible to practice the movements of *taijiquan* with such fullness without an intimate understanding of the martial implications, applications, and energy development. For example, one need never use splitting (one of the eight basic movements) to destroy an adversary's joints, but without understanding splitting, the movement will never be preformed correctly or mindfully. Without a clear understanding of splitting, there can be no mind intent or correct execution of this movement in the form. At best, this produces a diminished benefit, at worst, there is none. As Cheng Man-ch'ing explained, "*Taiji* form practice that ignores functional application bestows health benefits that are artificial at best."*

Another mistaken approach to *taijiquan* is assuming that those who are expert fighters also understand *taijiquan* because of this skill. Given the first reason why *taijiquan* is fading, searching for a "tough guy" as a teacher seems logical. While a clear demonstration of martial skill is an important qualifier for a teacher of any martial art, it cannot be the sole qualifying factor when choosing a teacher of *taijiquan*. The question is: does the teacher's martial skill come from his or her training in *taijiquan* or somewhere else?

The problem is that it has become very popular for the Chinese-style martial artist to

---

* See *Master Cheng's New Method of T'ai Chi Self-Cultivation*. Trans. Mark Hennessy.

study more than one style of martial art. Most hard stylists, those who practice an external type of martial art based in power from muscles instead of internal power (*shaolinquan* for example), take up *taijiquan* as a way to loosen up their joints and muscles and to improve their speed. They also benefit from the sensing skills learned in *taiji* push hands, one aspect of the two-person work of this system. Hard-style martial arts training often causes a great deal of injury to the body, so many take up *taijiquan* to heal themselves. So we come back to the misconceived approach to *taijiquan* as a health or exercise art.

The greatest difficulty in learning *taijiquan* is that the practitioner must completely relearn how to use the body from the outside in and the inside out. My teacher, Wang Yen-nien,[*] was already an accomplished martial artist when he was first introduced to his teacher of Yang Family *Michuan* style of *taijiquan*. Wang studied *shaolinquan, shuaijiao* (Chinese wrestling), and the internal arts of *xingyiquan* and *baguazhang* before deciding to include *taijiquan* in his repertoire. At the time, Master Wang was the hand-to-hand combat instructor at the military base where he was stationed, having mastered three systems of bayonet fighting. Upon meeting his future teacher, Zhang Qingling, the latter inquired as to what he had learned. After Master Wang stated all, the teacher refused to instruct him. Why? Wang would have to throw away all the *gongfu* he had accumulated in order to learn

---

[*] Wang Yen-nien of Shanxi province is my principle teacher. I study Yang Family *Michuan Taijiquan* and *Jin Shan Pai* Daoism under his guidance.

Taiji

taijiquan. Wang agreed to do so and was able to master *taijiquan*. The effort of overcoming years of external training was an amazing accomplishment.

We would expect that one martial art would lend to the next. This is true of training in more than one external art. Whichever art a student initially gains advanced skill in imprints the player with a particular understanding. All subsequent arts acquired will be learned and understood through that original framework. Simply stated, one who is skillful in the external martial arts, which employ muscle to develop power, will have a nearly impossible task of understanding *taijiquan*, which works in a completely different fashion, developing strength that comes from

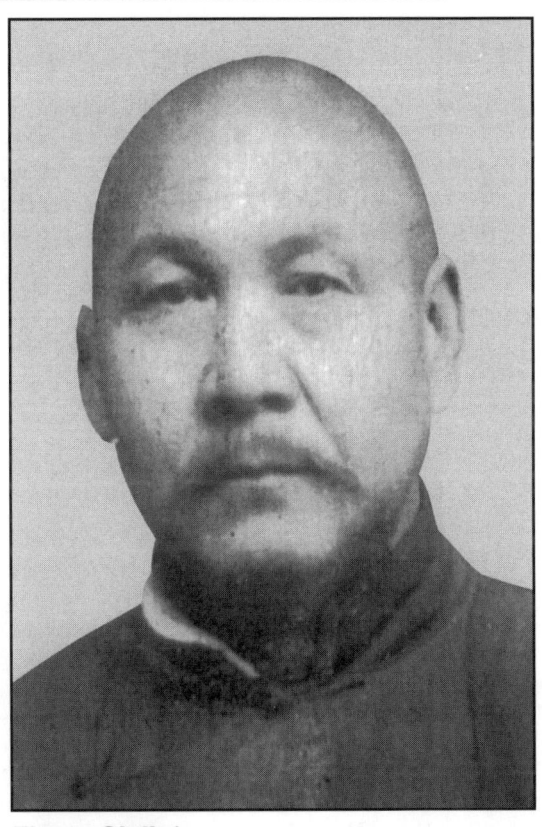

Zhang Qinlin*
1888-1967(?)

*Zhang Qingling was a student of Yang Jianhou and is famous as the last National Free Fighting Champion in China fought in the old way without rules or protective equipment. The Tournament was held in 1929, in Nanjing, which was China's Capitol at the time.

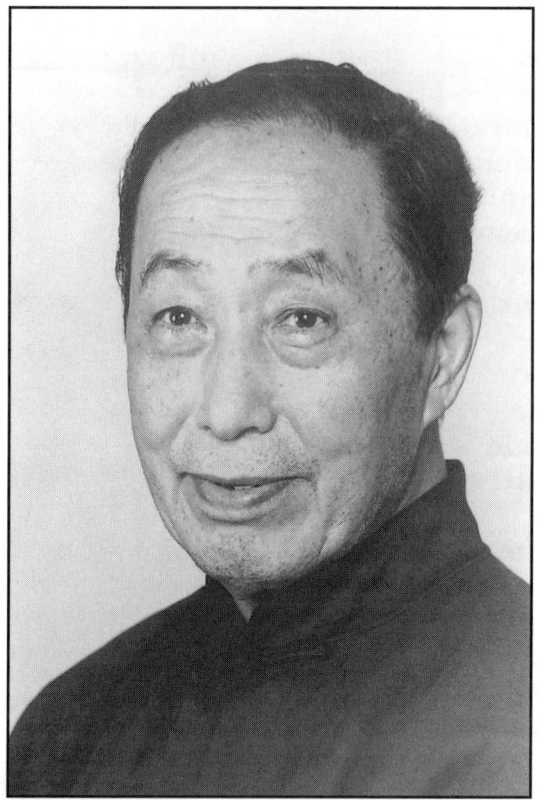

Wang Yen-nien
Born 1914

the ligaments and bones -- in other words, from the center outward.

Taijiquan is an art that works with the mind, body alignment, and *qi* in place of muscle development. Practitioners of external arts develop bodies that are literally hard, the muscles being toned hard from the exertion of repeatedly flexing them. The Yang families' writings on *taijiquan* clearly explain that the secret of their art is that it is "steel hidden in cotton," meaning, the strength is on the inside, and the muscles are soft, unclenched. Obviously, if a practitioner of an external martial art has spent years hardening his or her body, he or she cannot expect to then let all that muscle tension go and become soft. One simply cannot both train seriously at alternatively hardening and softening the body; these two practices are at cross-purposes.

Practitioners of hard styles might, indeed, have a thorough understanding of *taijiquan's* mechanics. They might even have a better understanding of these mechanics than those practicing *taijiquan* without its martial mind intent, as a "health art" only. However, internally their practice will not be *taijiquan*. When one of these hard stylists practices *taijiquan*, an advanced *taijiquan* student will be able to detect that the internal and external *jin* or intrinsic energy are not matched, that is the external movements of the body are not powered by energy or intent generated inside the body. This would indicate they are not practicing *taijiquan* from within. Unfortunately, several prominent Chinese *taijiquan* teachers today fall into this category.

Since nearly all good fighters today come from hard style schools (*taijiquan* is rarely taught as a fighting art, particularly in America), prospective students cannot simply search out the best fighters to teach them *taijiquan*, especially if that teacher has a history of, or is currently practicing, other arts.

To gain the benefits of *taijiquan*, whether our aim be modest (such as for health or stress reduction) or toward mastery, we must follow the path prescribed for us by the great masters of the art. For newcomers to decide that *taijiquan* (an art hundreds of years in development) can be altered in a few decades to fit their design or marketing needs is patently arrogant. Of all the masters whose instruction I have sought, those with the highest skill have changed nothing or very little from what their teachers taught them. The argument over adaptation ends there. Not only do these masters have all the benefits and skills that contemporary players are looking for, but also they are intelligent, witty people and the only ones truly qualified to make any changes in the system; yet they have clearly and mindfully chosen not to do so.

The System

Having established the most effective approach to *taijiquan,* we must now take a close look at the system itself. Most people think of the art as the slowly practiced movements of the empty-handed solo form. *Taijiquan* is actually an extensive system, as are most traditional martial arts. This is one manner in which *taijiquan* is similar to other Chinese martial arts.

What is most important to understand about *taijiquan* is that it is a system that is systematic. Each part of the system serves a specific purpose. And each purpose served feeds into the next part of the system. This feeding in or building of skills is not a simple, linear arrangement. There is also a process of development involving the body-mind, where more advanced parts of the system not only build upon skills previously learned but also draw out skills that are latent. These skills would be difficult to realize without the more advanced parts of the system. For this reason, it is important not only to practice the entire system, particularly if we are to reach a high level, but also to progress to each part at the right time and in the proper order. This is also an important reason why students of one system should not change or mix systems.

It is currently popular to study both the Yang and Chen Styles of *taijiquan* together. The idea is to learn the relaxed, soft nature from the Yang Style and to learn *fajin*, releasing energy, from the Chen. Students taking this path show both an ignorance of the method of *taijiquan* training -- that it is a system where new skills are introduced once a foundation for them has been established by previous training -- and of the Yang Style in particular. The Yang Style was created from the Chen Style and is a further development of the principles of *taijiquan*. The Yang Style solo form is more subtle than the Chen and, thus, can be employed to develop softness and mind intent to a greater degree. The Yang Style develops and trains *fajin* through the use of weapons* once the student's understanding and body has evolved sufficiently. A Chinese saying goes, "Chen Style is all steel, Yang Style is steel in cotton." This is not to say that the Chen style is not a complete system or that it is deficient in some way, but that each system has its own method of development.

The Yang family's *taijiquan* system is composed of basic exercises, the empty-handed solo form; *tuishou* (Push Hands), which can be further broken down into basic solo and two-person exercises, fixed-step *tuishou* (first single then two hands), and moving-step *tuishou*; *dalu*

*See my book, *Chinese Swordsmanship - The Yang Family Taiji Jian Tradition.*

The System

(cornering exercises); *sanshou* (free hands); and weapons training (traditional weapons include straight sword, saber, staff, and spear). As the practitioner evolves, developing each new skill, he will gradually add to his practice in the order presented here. He will also practice all the parts of the system he has learned, whether he is a beginner or an advanced swordsman.

Basic exercises work to open up

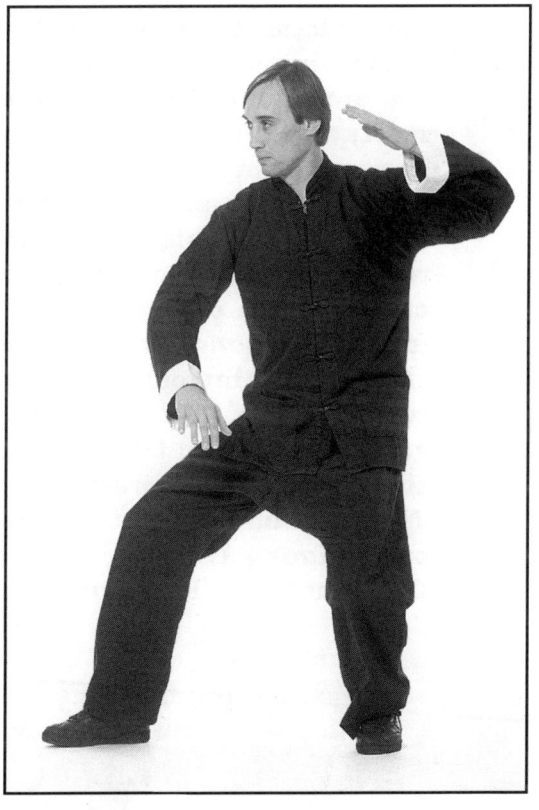

The author demonstrating the Brush Knee and Strike movement from the *Yangjia Michuan Taijiquan* form.

the body in ways specifically required by the mechanics of the various forms. These basic exercises also massage the internal organs and introduce the deep, diaphragmic breathing that, in coordination with the body movements, is a hallmark of *taijiquan*. It is important to realize how *taiji* basic exercises are different from either simple stretching or general Chinese systems of stretching exercises. While any type of stretching can be good for the body and *taijiquan*, *taiji* basic exercises are specifically designed to incorporate internal aspects of this art. This means that the *dantian* (one of the body's energy fields, located 1.3 inches below the navel) and the breath are employed from the start; a concentrated mind is involved from the beginning. In this way, *taiji* basic exercises can be thought of as a form of *qigong* or "energy work" though this is not a traditional term. (The reader should note that while *taijiquan* has been called a form of *qigong*, it is not. *Taijiquan* is a form of *neigong*, literally "internal work." A later treatise will introduce the importance of *neigong* to relaxation. *Qigong* is a term currently being generally applied to all forms of internal exercise that involve deep breathing or *qi* in any fashion. This is a modern, not traditional, use of the term *qigong* as promoted by the Chinese Communists. The Communists wish to downplay

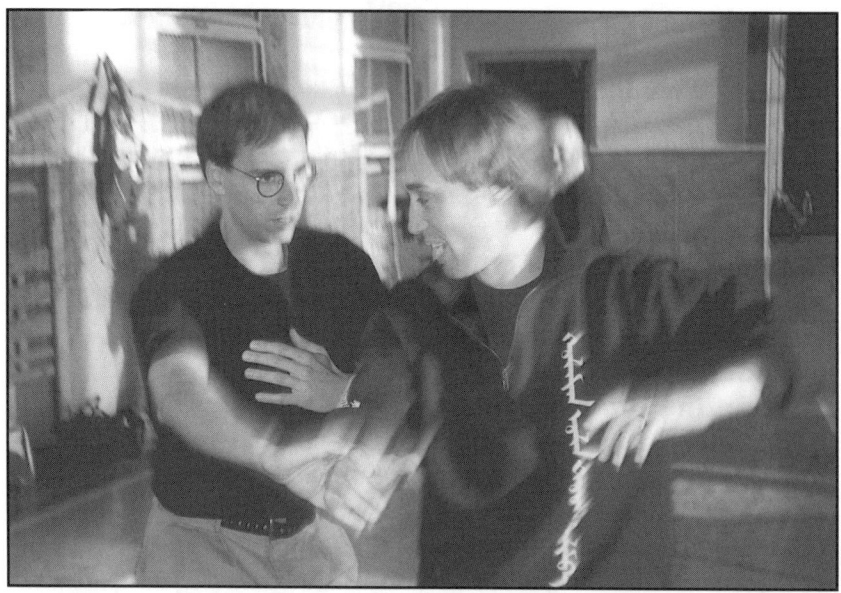

The author and a senior student enjoying some full-power, full-speed *tuishou* after a seminar in Tallinn, Estonia.

The System

the Daoist influence in the creation of these systems and the metaphysics that go along with them.)

The solo form cultivates specific conditions in the body while developing proper mechanics that allow for the release of muscle tension, enhance *qi* flow, and allow for self-defense. Some principles of movement the form cultivates include (1) that all movements are controlled and directed by the waist, (2) the muscles are released of tension, allowing them to become loose and soft (*fang song*),* (3) the torso is "suspended" with the spine vertical, and (4) the weight is "separated" so that at no time is the body weight distributed equally in the feet when the movement is being applied.

Tuishou (push hands) begins putting the mechanics of the form into practice. Push Hands develops the skills for *ting* (listening), *dong* (understanding), *hua* (deflecting) and *fajin* (releasing energy), amongst others. Push hands training, thus, provides the student with a step-by-step learning environment for applying the mechanics acquired in the solo form, combined with the principles of yielding, neutralizing, and releasing. Naturally, each step of push hands training becomes increasingly more difficult as both the level of the players increases along with the complexity of the exercises. The skills of push hands can, then, be married to the mechanics of the solo form for *sanshou* (free hands). Push hands and free hands move the basic idea underlying *taijiquan*, staying calm and relaxed in body-mind at all times, from the

*see the treatise on *fang song* below.

conceptual world to the real world. By learning to stay calm, loose, soft, and focused in these controlled physical conflicts, we can more easily see and confront our own aggression and tension. From there, the practitioner gradually learns to let go, become soft, and be free from tension. Then he/she can move to dealing with the more common types of conflicts experienced in the workplace and home.

Weapons forms are more difficult than the empty-hand solo form. They help advance the skills learned in empty-hand practice. Practicing with weapons strengthens the body, and, thus, the spirit. Specifically, weapons provide a device into which to *fajin* (release energy) within the framework of a form. Naturally, releasing energy can be learned during push hands training, but a weapons form provides the context in which to practice a specific movement or technique over and over, thus allowing for refinement of this skill. It is also easier to *fajin* into a sword or long weapon because neither the steel nor wood will soften and learn how to yield. In short, weapons are the perfect practice partner for training *fajin*. Each weapon has a different attribute and trains the body to *fajin* in different manners. For example, the *dao* (saber) chops in a heavy, axe-like fashion; the *jian* (straight sword) employs precise cuts and thrusts; and the *chiang* (spear) and *dagan* (long stick) develops thrusting and coiling with expanding movements and are the most physically demanding weapons.

The System within the System

    Many masters have set down *taiji* principles. Yang Chengfu* recorded twelve points, Cheng Man-ch'ing** derived five principles, and Wang Yen-nien gives us eight. Each was describing the same thing. Each came up with a set of principles, or more accurately "pieces," that describe the whole. We need these principles because we do not have a single word that means all of them at once. Yet even though we divide up *taijiquan* into principles, it remains one whole. No principle exists on its own, and each principle is important to the development of the next. The converse is also true. A weakness in one principle will retard the others.

---

*See *Tai Chi Touchstones: Yang Family Secret Transmissions*, trans. Douglas Wile, for a list of Yang Chenfu's principles.

**See *Cheng Tzu's Thirteen Treatises on T'ai Chi Ch'uan*, trans. Ben Lo, for a list of Cheng Man-ch'ing's principles.

20

Slow

Slow movement is one of the distinguishing characteristics of *taijiquan*. No other martial art employs this method of training as does ours. However, many mistake simply moving slowly for practicing *taijiquan*. Clearly, taking a *shaolinquan* set and practicing it slowly would not make it *taijiquan*. The movements of *taijiquan* must follow the principles set down in "the classics",* no matter what speed a form is practiced at. Moving slowly through any set of movements will certainly bring about a sense of relaxation as any slowing down from our normal pace would. But this sense of relief and even fluidity is just as certainly not *taijiquan*. Moving slowly alone does not make *taijiquan*.

Students must stop and ask why -- not to question or challenge a teacher's authenticity -- but to understand how each portion of the training works with the others and what principles

---
* There are a number of literary transmissions from past masters of *taijiquan* that are generally referred to as "the classics." See Selected Readings.

are to be learned from it. Why practice the movements slowly?

It was William C.C. Chen* who truly opened my eyes to the meaning of slow movement. We were sitting in a donut shop after class, discussing *sanshou* (Free Hands) training. Chen always began a student's *sanshou* training with two students practicing boxing at the pace they practice the form while wearing standard professional 16 oz. gloves. When I inquired why, Chen answered "we practice *taijiquan* slowly" and then paused, allowing my thought "This is a surprise?" to pass. Then he finished his answer -- "and precise." If new students began sparring at even a slightly increased speed, nervousness would turn it into an all-arms slugfest, devoid of any proper principles of *taijiquan*.

Learning *taijiquan* means completely relearning how to use the body. Practicing slowly creates the opening for precision. Initially in *taijiquan*, a student must work on cleanness and precise articulation of movement. I once asked a group of beginners why we practiced slowly. One student who played piano replied, "When studying a difficult piece of music, I practice it slowly so that I can correct the mistakes as they happen." She is absolutely correct. Slowness allows time for an awareness of the body to manifest and for the practitioner to act on this awareness. Take, for instance, *fang song*, literally meaning "let loose and unclench the muscles" (this process is discussed in detail in the essay begin-

---

* Master Chen has been teaching in New York City since the 1960's. He was Zheng Manqing's youngest disciple, nicknamed the "Little Master."

Slow

ning on page 27). The first, important step in releasing muscle tension is proper body alignment. Without correct alignment, *fang song* is not possible. This is because one's muscle tension is in part a result of misalignment; this tension is required for holding the body in its misaligned state. Once a student has achieved a minimum level of proper alignment, his body is free to work as a single unit with a precision that was not possible before.

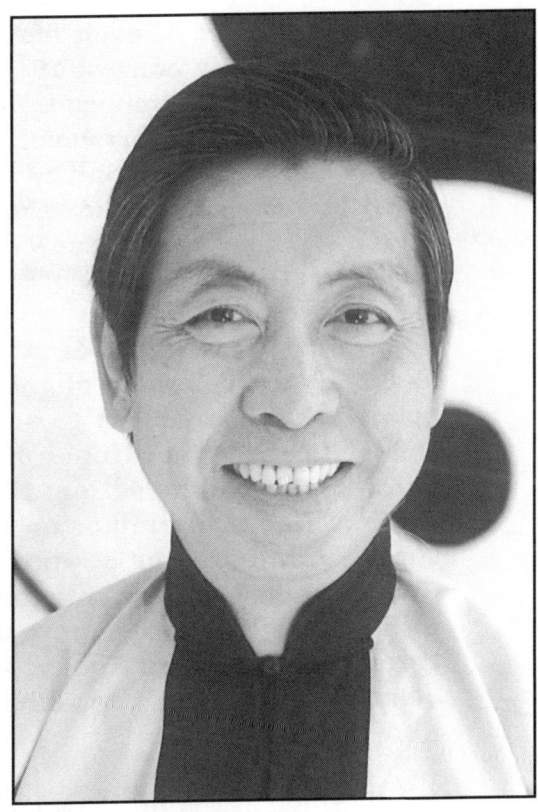

William C. C. Chen
Born 1935

Reaching a condition where the correct body alignment alone maintains the body structure without significant muscle tension takes several years of practice. And it is a process that deepens over years and decades. But once a basic level of alignment is achieved, the mind can focus on deeper elements of the form, and "slowness" takes on added meaning.

Freed from tension through correct alignment, the body can begin to truly follow the breath. The pace of each movement may have been dictated by control of the breath earlier, but this pace was imposed. Being loose and soft, even on an elementary level, opens the way to letting the body ride on the breath. The classics instruct: "The mind leads the *qi*, and the *qi* leads the body." The mind-intent's ability to lead the *qi* is directly related to controlled breathing.

Just as slowness of movement allows for a new body awareness of alignment, going slow will now allow for an ability to see internally. With this sight, the practitioner discovers the *dantian* and its bellows-like action. Next, one uncovers the *mai* (inner meridians or vessels the *qi* moves through) and breaths down to the *Yong Chuan* (Bubbling Well point). This process continues until all eight *mai* open, circulating the *qi* throughout the entire body. This is what the classics describe as threading the pearl with the nine-crooked paths.

Slowness is no longer merely a means for learning the basics. Slow movement is the joy of meditation. The *taijiquan* form becomes a vessel for concentration meditation, for inner work (*neigong*). "The *dantian* is like a bank where we store *qi*. When we need it, we can bring it out," says Master Wang Yen-nien.

Flow

Flow

    Flow is a sign of progress in *taijiquan*. Speaking of flow within the form brings to mind images from the classics, such as "*Changquan** flows on unceasingly" and "Move like a great river." The feeling is of unceasing movement, perpetual motion, constancy.

    Flow is not only a sign of advancement. It must be cultivated throughout years of practice. Flow ultimately is the bringing together of all the body's parts. Flow is the elimination of the parts. Or more correctly, flow is the realization that there are no parts, just one harmonious whole. Flow is the absence of obstacles.

    Lack of flow means rips and tears in the practice. This has implications on a number of levels. In relation to the health aspects, it means that the *qi* flow is not continuous or even. Without flow, the *qi* may possibly even stagnate if the breath is being held tightly at the "tear" or

---

* *Changquan* is an old name for *taijiquan*, which literally means "long boxing" or "fist." *Chang* can also be taken to mean "to flow without end."

the break in the flow of movement (a common beginner's error). Concerning self-defense, a tear in the flow is an opening, a stop that the *duifang* (one's "opposite," -- see page 39 for a full discussion of this term) will take advantage of. In respect to meditation, the concentration of the *yi* (mind) has been broken and is possibly lost.

    The break in mind has the greatest implications. When there is not flow, there is dead space. It is not a void with the implications of creation but is a dead, mindless space, or, in other words, not mindful. A dead space is not being in the present. It is not being present here in this moment. *Taijiquan*, as a Daoist-influenced art, strives to bring the practitioner into present moment awareness. Present moment awareness, being absolutely in each movement, in each moment of each movement, without severance or break, is the enlightened state of *taijiquan*. It is one small step that can be made towards the mystical aspects of the art.

Fang Song

"Let the mind direct the *qi* so that it sinks deeply and steadily and permeates the bones."

Wang Chung Yueh,
Mental Elucidation of the Thirteen Postures

To discuss the idea and method of *fang song* -- literally "let loose and unclench the muscles" -- we must understand that it is not an end. *Fang song* is not something we escape to, finding refuge from life's stress and pain. *Fang song* is the Way -- a Way in which it becomes difficult for an attacker to find a hard place to strike and harm us, a Way where pain and stress find little to land on. We learn the Way of *fang song* through the body, but it speaks to our whole being. (It should be noted that although *fang song* is most typically translated as "relaxed," I feel this is at best misleading and is an inaccurate translation.)

The one truly unique element to *taijiquan*

that separates it from all other martial arts is its way of cultivating and using the body. The Chinese term for this is *fang song*. There are no words in English which have the same meaning as *fang song*.

Fang means to be loose, let loose or be loose fitting. *Song* means soft, unclenched muscle, while implying looseness. For years, I approached *fang song* as "dynamic relaxation" (whatever that was supposed to mean) as something I had to do. Practicing the form, I was "doing" my *fang song*. Many American students of Cheng Man-ch'ing said that when asked how to *fang song* he said, "let go." When asked how to "let go," he replied, "relax." The master's answers seemed a paradox, the type of paradox that drives beginners mad -- that is, until we begin to examine the method of *fang song* and the more exact meaning of the words *fang song*.

Fang is to let loose and *song* to unclench and soften the muscles. Feeling soft and, thus, relaxed, it is easy to release tension, to let loose. There is nothing one needs to do to reach *song* in the *taiji* form or life. It is not even a matter of undoing; it is a matter of not doing -- of not doing tension, of not doing muscular force. Consciously reducing the amount of muscular force used when practicing the form is the first, vital step in developing a deeper, more dynamic state of *fang song*. The more *song* (soft), the greater *fang* (releasing, loosening, letting go). Cheng's paradox is, in truth, instruction.

These simple insights point to a more important truth of *taijiquan*. The whole process is continuous, step by step. A common misconception in *taijiquan* is that by diligently practicing the form a certain magical number of rounds (some where in the neighborhood of 36,000), the immortals will shine a divine, golden light down from heaven, and the worthy disciple will be transformed into a master of extraordinary ability. This does not even happen in comic books.

The first step in developing *fang song* is proper body structure and alignment. Once this is achieved, even in an elementary manner, much less muscle tension is needed to hold the body up. The student has simply learned how to use the body more efficiently. This allows an active letting go of muscle tension that was needed to balance the body's old misalignments. Previous to proper alignment, the body was leaning this way and that, the spine curved in ways that threw one off balance, the head was always tilted forward, etc. Tense muscles acted as guide wires, holding the body in place like a stiff tower. Once aligned, the weight of the body falls vertically into the feet, nailing one straight down. The tension guide wires are no longer necessary.

As less tension is required to support the body and movement, an opportunity is created. The mind is employed to let go of muscular tension. This experience teaches the student just how to let go. In letting go, two important results are achieved. The first is that the practitioner experiences the strength of body, a seemingly effortless strength, that arrives without tension and that the body can express power without tension. And, second, now that some of the tension is out of the way, it is that much easier to listen to the body and to better align it.

The result is a natural progression where even more tension guide wires are released. Cheng's advice, "let go to relax and relax to let go," now finds its place.

Many have discovered this process and left tension behind. Eventually, this process slows and reaches the apparent end. The practitioner has released all the guide wires that were unnecessary, that is all those created by misalignment. However, a few remain, and these cannot be cut. This remaining tension cannot be eliminated because there must be some strength, something solid in the body, to hold it up. For most *taijiquan* practitioners today, there is a missing link to developing internal strength: *qi*. Yet the classics point at the method, and they give us a ruler by which to measure masters. The body of an advanced *taijiquan* practitioner is described as "steel wrapped in cotton." These classics explain that the mind directs the *qi*, which directs the body. Working to develop the mind-intent to direct the flow of *qi* develops an internal strength that can take the place of muscle strength.

Many contemporary *taijiquan* students, lacking a background in Daoism, have turned to *qigong* for their internal development. This is a good, educated guess but unfortunately misses the mark. *Qigong* practices, inspired by Daoists, have taken myriad forms. Over the millennia, new forms of *qigong* were developed in response to different needs. Doctors of traditional Chinese medicine developed forms of *qigong* (and other exercises, such as the Five Animal Frolics) as a means of physical therapy and as treatments for specific conditions. These doctors could prescribe a specific type of *qigong* to treat a certain imbalance that was causing a patient to be sick, either in conjunction with other treatment or alone. Many health-oriented types of *qigong* were also developed as health tonics. Many types of *qigong* were likewise developed by Buddhists to augment their meditation practice. Buddhist methods of spiritual cultivation do not involve *qi*. Therefore, their interest in *qi* is limited to simple body strengthening.

The thousands of forms of *qigong* that have been developed over the centuries (currently over 3,000 types have been cataloged in Mainland China) have retained this simplified or specialized nature. (*Neigong*, in comparison, is a deeper meditative practice and is, in fact, the Daoist manner of personal cultivation). Each type of *qigong* has a mind-intent specific to its goals. Accordingly, the reason why we cannot graft any handy form of *qigong* available into our *taijiquan* is that this art also has specific goals and, thus, uses a specific mind-intent and method of *qi* cultivation. The fact that this mixing of arts has become commonplace speaks to the fragmentary nature of the transmission of *taijiquan* in the last hundred years.

Through the process of *fang song,* we feel and experience the most basic Daoist principle underlying *taijiquan*. *Yin* (softness) gives rise to *yang* (hardness); the greater the *yin*, the greater the *yang*. The more softness we develop in the body through tension release, the more we relax. The softer, more *song* the body/mind is, the more natural and easy it is for the *qi* to flow and, thus, permeate and strengthen the bones, making them steel-like.

Softness also translates into *fajin* (releasing energy) power (see the next chapter for an in-depth discussion of *fajin*). As a soft body becomes springy and whip-like, it can transfer power from the body's foundation in the feet and legs through the spine and out the hands. Less tension (read softness) means less in the way of the wave of *fajin* from the root. This translates to more energy released through the hands. Again, the greater softness, *yin*, produces the greater power or hardness, *yang*.

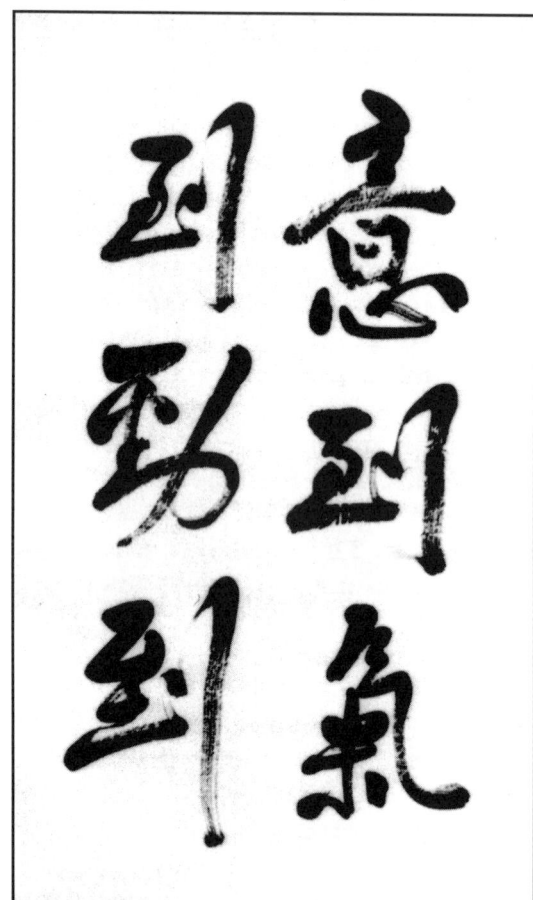

"Mind Arrives,
Qi Arrives,
Power Arrives."
calligraphy by Ben Lo

Breathing & *Fajin*

The importance of proper breathing cannot be overstated. Breathing with and into movements is precisely what makes the form more than a series of mere body movements. Coordinating the breath with the movements is what makes *taijiquan neigong*.

The *Taiji* Classic, *Exposition of Insights into the Thirteen Postures*, by Wu Yuxiang clearly instructs us to "[u]se mind intent (*xin*) to move *qi*. Make the *qi* calmly sink, so that it can soak into the bones. Use the *qi* to move the body" (author's translation). With each movement, one whole breath - inhale, exhale - is completed. In Daoist arts, breathing is referred to as *tuna*.* *Tuna* is written with two characters. *Tu* means to let go and *na* to grab or draw back in. The idea is more than simply breathing in and out, including releasing and drawing back into the center as parts of a whole. There is an implicit intent in the term *tuna*. When inhaling during the beginning of each movement, the *qi*

* In spoken Chinese, *xiho* is used for breathing, literally meaning "inhale, exhale."

is drawn in by the *dantian* down along the *ren mai* (which runs down the front of the torso) and down the inside of legs into the *yong chuan*, bubbling well, point in the foot. (The *yong chuan* point is located in the center of the foot, right behind the ball of the foot at the same location as the Kidney meridian 1 point.) The mind concentrates, and, thus, the *qi* is concentrated into the foot that carries most of the body weight. With exhalation, the energy stored in the "root" and *dantian* are released and directed upward through the legs and into the *du mai* (which lies along the spine). With each breath, not only is inhalation and exhalation completed but also the *qi* is moved through one complete turn.
Touching the tongue to the palate connects the *ren* and *du mai* so that the circuit can be completed. Being able to move the *qi* naturally up and down the body is the first step toward using *qi* to mobilize and support the body. (The directions given here are for men; women circulate *qi* in the opposite direction.)

William C.C. Chen will tell you that when striking, your mind should be in whichever part of the body is connecting with the *duifang*. This might surprise many *taijiquan* practitioners. When practicing the form, all beginners are taught to concentrate on the *dantian*. The task of perching the mind on this single point seems at first enough work for a lifetime. I asked Master Chen about this apparent discrepancy and what Cheng Man-ch'ing had taught. Chen explained that the first step is to get the mind in the *dantian*. From there, the mind is sunk down into the *yong chuan* points in the feet and, next, up the legs into the spine. Once this is achieved, the arms are added to the circula-

Breathing & *Fajin*

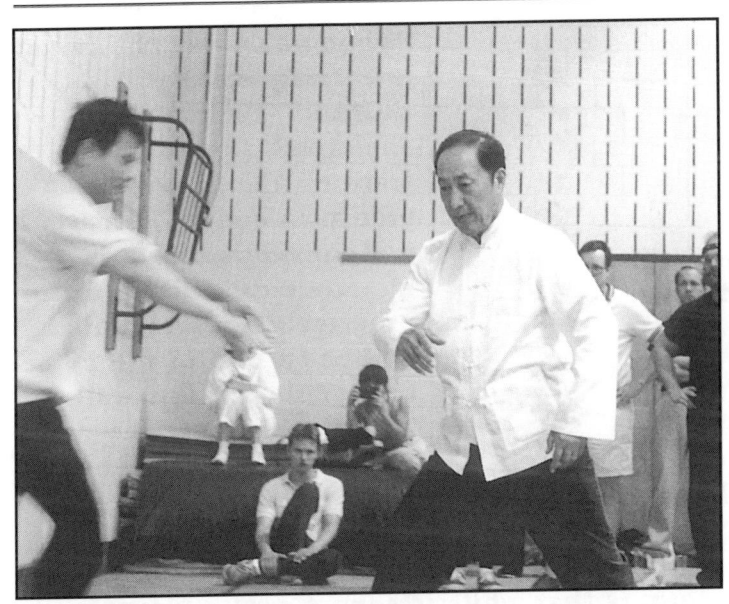

Wang Yen-nien demonstrating *peng* (wardoff) *fajin* at a Great River Taoist seminar, 1988.

tion, and the mind is also sent into the tiger and dragon points in the palms. Concentrating on the *dantian* alone is for beginners. Advanced practitioners concentrate on the *dantian*, the points in the feet and hands, and the *baihui* on top of the head. Essentially, the mind is aware of and connecting all these points throughout the entire body through the unified flow of mind and *qi* along the meridians.

After a few years' practice, I connected the complete circuit, but I wondered how to use or release *qi* during *fajin*. Circulating the *qi* around the body is not difficult with practice, but it is slow, moving at the pace of the form. *Fajin* is said to be released like an arrow from a bow. One doesn't strike or push at form speed. I couldn't see being able to move my *qi* that fast along the meridians to *fajin*. I spoke with Wang Yen-nien about this point, and his words added to what I had learned from Chen years before:

"Root in the Foot, Explode from the leg." Signed William C.C. Chen, presented to the author at a Great River Taoist seminar.

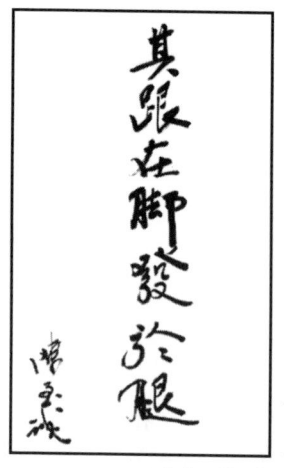

"When you *fajin*, the mind is entirely on the *duifang*," the master explained. Don't concentrate on the *qi* moving in your own body. The path and movement of *qi* is already natural from form practice. Focus the mind and body, and *qi* will come out. "The *dantian* is like a bank: everyday you put in a little so that it is there when you need to bring it out," Wang explained.

One of the interesting aspects of using *qi* to *fajin* is that while it's more powerful and faster, something your training partner will attest to, it does not feel "stronger" to you because there is less and less muscle tension. We usually associate strength with the tension we feel when using our muscles. When we have lifted something quite heavy, there is a lot of tension in the arms, and we feel that we are strong. The strength of *fajin* is not experienced in the same way. Instead, one feels a rush of *qi* up the body as you *fajin*.

Every practitioner must strengthen the mind and increase his or her *qi* so that it goes everywhere in the body. Circulating the *qi* in this way nourishes the body. Circulating the *qi* in this fashion also causes the *qi* to slowly permeate the bones, strengthening them.

Proper breathing alone does not create great *taijiquan*, but without it, the form remains empty.

Basics

Beginners are always anxious to finish the basics and get on to the more exciting, advanced teachings. Advanced students are always happy working the basics.

• • •

There is an American archer who is, perhaps, the greatest archer living at this time. Aside from being the Olympic Champion, he was champion of nearly every other tournament, whether indoors or out. At the height of his career, his scores started dropping. No one could imagine his scores doing anything except increase. How did he regain his high marks? By making the most elementary basic correction for all martial arts: he corrected his stance by first getting his feet in the proper position. Then, he marked that position with chalk. Every time it was his turn to shoot, he placed his feet in the marked positions.

• • •

Once I attended *tuishou* training with Ray Haywood, a senior student of T.T. Liang. The morning session was very instructive, focusing on two-hand *tuishou* (push hands) techniques. An advanced class was also planned for the afternoon. Excited by the morning's workout, I looked forward to learning still more two-hand techniques to improve my *tuishou*. But when the class started, we began with simple, single-hand circling. In fact, the entire advanced class dealt with basic, single-hand *tuishou* training. Halfway through the session, Haywood stopped and related a story about a friend of his who was fifth *dan* Gojo Ryu Karateka. He asked his friend, "Do you still practice basic drills?" The Karateka replied, "Do you think when I do them they're basic?"

I have never given up basic, single-hand *tuishou* training, and I credit it with much of my tournament success in later years.

• • •

A classmate of mine returned to Taiwan one summer to study intensively with Master Wang Yen-nien. Arriving early enough every morning to stretch out before the beginning of the 6:00 am class, one of his most profoundly motivating experiences was to look up one morning and see Wang stretching his legs too. He realized he had seen the Master there everyday when he arrived, practicing this most simple basic thing. (Wang Yen-nien was in his seventies at the time and rated as a ninth degree teacher by the National *T'ai Chi Ch'uan* Association.)

Duifang

There is absolutely no word in the English language for the Chinese term *duifang*. There is no corresponding idea in Western martial terminology. *Duifang*, used throughout the classics, is most often translated as "opponent." This immediately gives the wrong feeling. An opponent is someone who exists in an adversarial position; he or she is an obstacle. We think of our adversaries as enemies. Enemies are people we grow to hate. The notion of an opponent easily manifests as resistance and stiffness in mind and body.

Duifang literally means the "other direction." We could ask who was "*duifang*" to you at dinner (meaning who sat across from you). The idea of two-person work in *taijiquan* is that of a lever, a balance. As on an old-fashion scale where two pans are balanced on opposite sides of a beam, in this art's two-person work, two students stand opposite each other but are joined. The classic "Song of Push Hands" explains that there is no idea of separation. *Taijiquan* is all "no resistance and no letting go," all stick, adhere, follow.

Wang Yen-nien demonstrating *lu* (rollback) at a Great River Taoist seminar, 1988.

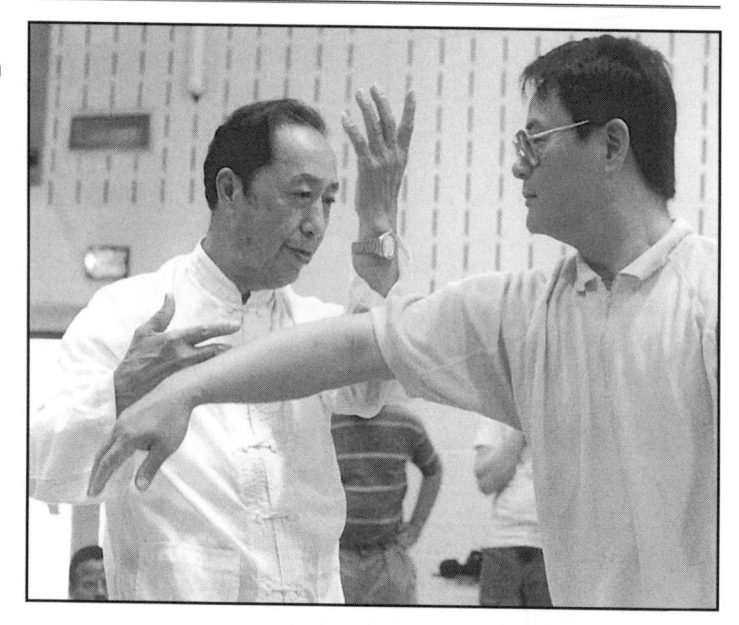

When one's *duifang* - opposite direction - pushes into the center, one turns, yielding in exact proportion to the push, leading it off center. As the push is slipping off the center, the side of one's body that is opposite the side that is yielding swings like a lever toward the *duifang* and circularizes the incoming energy. This is how the rollback* movement is applied, deflecting the *duifang's* push before it arrives. When using rollback or any other movement, there is no thought of using the rollback technique. Rollback is what the *duifang* asked for.

Duifang implies listening, joining, and blending. There is an appropriateness about techniques that manifest through soft sticking and following. Correctly applied, *taijiquan* never over-reacts or pulls away and never forces techniques.

* Rollback is one of *taijiquan's* eight basic movements.

Tuishou - Ting Jin, Dong Jin, Hua Jin

"[The serious student] cannot use techniques of softness - he must become soft, 'the very atoms in his body must relax.' Then his *taijiquan* will start to work."
Wolfe Lowenthal,
There are No Secrets

Tuishou practice has many implications. Though it seems to merely train martial reflexes, *tuishou* can have a profound effect on life. *Tuishou* training begins with sensing, referred to in Chinese as *ting jin*. *Ting jin* literally means "listening energy," though sensitivity is developed first through and in the hands. A *taijiquan* player develops *ting jin* to "hear" the *duifang's* structure, his or her very bones, with the lightest touch. From this "listening," a player knows what is happening in the *duifang*. Is the *duifang* relaxed and calm, is his or her body (mind) tense and rigid or even frozen, or tense like a spring ready to pop? Is the *duifang* centered and balanced or falling off balance before he or she even

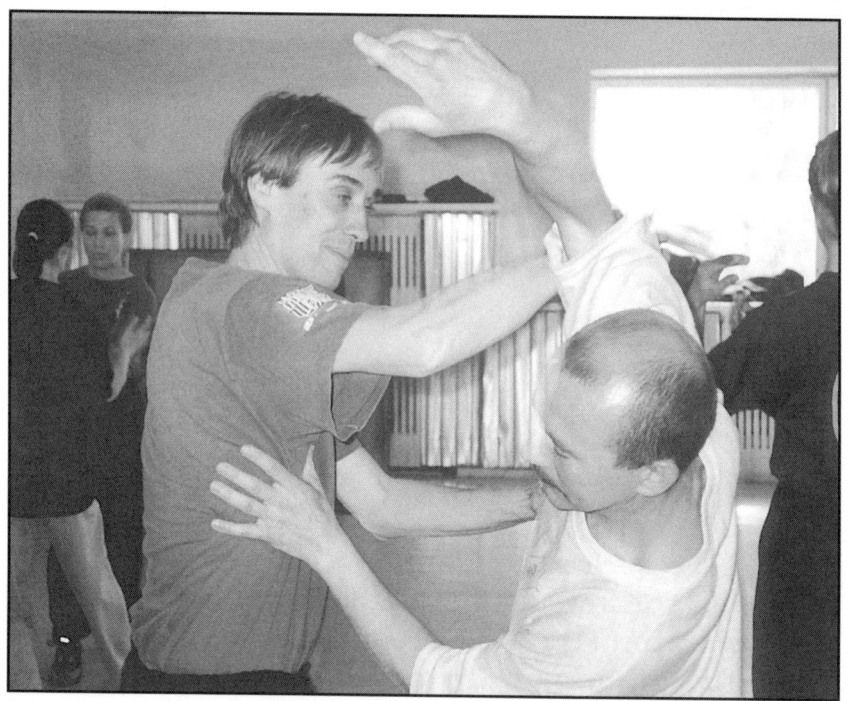

The author playing *tuishou* with a senior student in Narva, Estonia.

moves? The "listener" also senses the location of the *duifang's* center, connecting with it softly so that the *duifang* is unaware of the joining. Waiting alert, the advanced player is ready to circularize any attack, yielding and neutralizing the incoming force while at the exact same time using the moment of that force to move in on the *duifang's* center and push him or her out.

Next, *dong jin*, literally "interpreting or understanding energy," is developed. Closely related to *ting jin*, *dong jin* is knowing the meaning of what is "heard," interpreting *ting jin*. *Ting jin* is a musical code; *dong jin* is understanding the message. Before the *duifang* is able to manifest his/her energy, the *taijiquan* player knows where it is going.

Tuishou

With an understanding of the *duifang's* attack, the next step is clear: applying *hua jin*, deflecting energy. The *duifang's* energy can be led off-center while not exposing one's own structure, which remains concealed in softness. Employing the technique rollback (*lu*), one can deflect the energy of the *duifang's* attack so that it falls into a void. The advanced player uses "four ounces to deflect a thousand pounds." Only four ounces are required through knowing or intuiting the precise place and moment to deflect. "By following our *duifang's* position we can achieve the marvelous effect of transforming energy or deflecting energy," explains Cheng Man-ch'ing in his record of Yang Chengfu's Twelve Important Points. The energy can also be bounced back into the *duifang's* center, taking him or her off balance, with wardoff (*peng*). With the *duifang* now neutralized and his or her center known, one can choose whether one wants to *fajin*, release energy, and how much power to employ. Whether employing *lu* (rollback) or *peng* (wardoff) to deflect, the response must be appropriate to the incoming energy, or one's intention will be exposed and countered.

When beginners try their hands at *tuishou*, they typically overreact. Pulling away replaces yielding. Shoving with arm muscles is substituted for *fajin*. Listening degrades into nervous reflex reactions. Beginners approximate the outside, playing techniques instead of developing internally. It is easy for *tuishou* between beginners to turn into a shoving match, resembling schoolyard wrestling. Beginners see their practice partners as people to overcome. They break the balance by resisting and not following; there is no *duifang*; there is an opponent.

Working with an advanced player quickly reminds beginners of the powerful nature of softness. When pulling away to avoid incoming energy instead of yielding, momentum is created; a tendency to fall manifests in the body. The *duifang* will follow this path and adds to it when the body runs out of run-away room. Seemingly out of nowhere, a push appears and, with little energy applied, one flies away, off balance.

Beginners lose the balance between themselves and the *duifang* until they internalize *ting jin*, *dong jin*, and *hua jin*. Approximating the outward techniques comes out as overreaction. As principle evolves and mechanical focus on technique recedes, an appropriateness appears. A balance is formed. Reflex gives way to sensitivity.

Sensitivity in the game of push hands creates the possibility for sensitivity out on the street. In *tuishou*, we let the *duifang* push with as much power as he or she likes but offer no place for him or her to push. We take away his or her target. The body seems outwardly as cotton, as a cloud. Softness hides the inner strength. Listening informs us if a push is for the center or missing. Making a small adjustment with the waist and legs, one removes the target, and the *duifang's* push finds nothing to lean on.

What evolves in the body will evolve in the mind, attitude, and psyche if one lets it. When "facing an opponent" has been transformed into "joining with the *duifang*," a fight and struggle no longer exists. Only the resolution of balance remains.

Sanshou

Sanshou (literally "free hands") was once widely practiced by the founders of *taijiquan* and their students. Of the first three generations of the Yang family, all were known for their outstanding martial skill. In the Yang family *Michuan Taijiquan* lineage, Zhang Qinlin, student of Yang Jianhou, was famous for besting all comers in the Chinese National Fighting Tournament of 1929. Of Zhang, Wang Yen-nien said, "No one could last more than four or five blows with him."

Today, *taijiquan* is practiced far from the crucible of the Chinese battlefield where it developed. (It should be kept in mind that the Yang family made their living as military trainers during a time of rampant warfare. The city where they were employed to train the militia was besieged three times during the Taiping Rebellion.) So, in some ways, it is not surprising that few practice or develop the martial aspects of our art, though this is clearly encouraged by the writings of the Yang family.

More the pity is that *sanshou* has become a dirty word in many *taijiquan* circles. *Sanshou* is branded as violent and counterproductive. Some even go so far as to say that teaching "self-defense" is improper because it teaches students that they have a "self" to protect. Putting philosophy aside, there really is a naiveté to such statements. As a teacher with women students, some of whom have been raped and beaten, I have seen the emotional and physical scars of such attacks. For me, it is far more immoral to withhold the tools of "self-defense" from those good people when they have asked for them than it is to risk some misunderstanding in training. After all, we live in the real world, not on some mountaintop. I can assure you, being brutalized does not aid students on any spiritual quest. More telling is that such negative criticism of *sanshou* is only made by those who have not practiced it. For myself and my students, the more we have learned from *sanshou*, the more we have embraced it. Practically speaking, several of my women and men students escaped attackers on the street unscathed by using simple techniques they learned in class. However, if they had not engaged in *sanshou* training to complement their form application training, they would not have remained calm enough on the street to apply these simple techniques.

Contrary to the general misconception held by the uninitiated, proper practice of *taiji sanshou* does not lead to a more aggressive or violent person. In fact, in my personal experience and from what I have seen in my students, the result is exactly the opposite. I have watched the frightened, the aggressive, and the

Sanshou

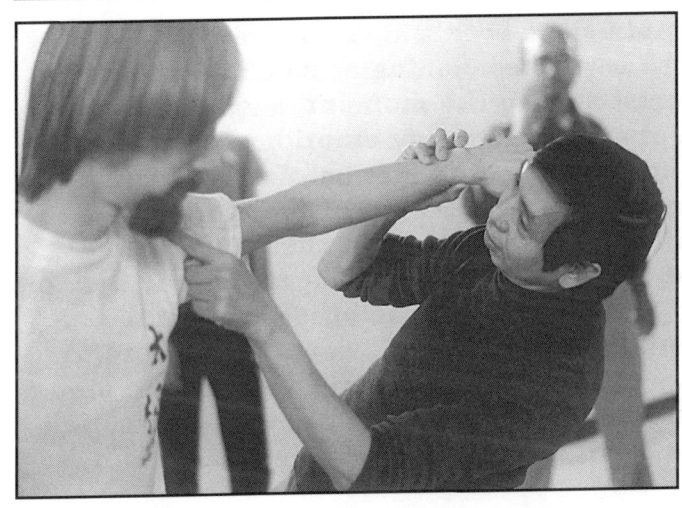

William C.C. Chen explaining the fine points of striking to the author at a Great River Taoist Center seminar, 1986.

unconfident evolve into people free from the inhibitions created by those emotions. More than one student who began training with a bad temper and with an urge to hit first ended up a confident, stable person who left behind violent urges.

Key to this personal evolution is the correct approach to practicing *sanshou* as "free hands," not sparring and most certainly not as fighting. In *taijiquan*, there is no blocking, and the *duifang's* force is never impeded or fought against. Rather, any incoming strike or kick is redirected in such a way that it is changed.

This is not a simple matter of "going with the flow," being tossed wherever the current drags you. For me, this does not feel any different than skiing down a steep mountain, canoeing down rapids, or even listening to Mozart. It is using the current to get where you want to go. In *sanshou*, the only difference is it is not the flow of the river's current or shape of the mountain slope with which I am moving, but the pattern of strikes coming at me. To achieve this, you must stay in the moment, a goal of every form of meditation. Any emotions or thoughts that occur during the stream of strikes coming at you takes you right out of the moment. They are like big, jagged rocks in the rapids. Being afraid of what is going to happen to your nose or what you might do to the other guy's nose is a self-fulfilling prophecy. As soon as you stop to think, you are stopped. Just like trying to stop and suddenly stand up straight while skiing full speed down a steep, snow-covered mountain, you fall.

I cannot tell you the number of times I have been punched in the nose while playing *sanshou* with one of my beginner students. It happens every time I stop and think about what correction I need to give them. It does not matter how much greater my skill is than theirs. If I am not in the moment, I am just a target.

The process of learning *sanshou* is very simple. Take the experience of yielding and releasing power from *tuishou*, marry it to the good mechanics of the form, and just start playing. Inevitably, everyone learning *sanshou* will get bruises and more. That is not important. Sticking with training will get you to an unbruisable place. When I began *sanshou* training, I had lots of bruises on my forearms from blocking instead of using rollback. I had no one to blame but myself for them. As the number grew less and less with practice, I took that as a measure of my progress until, at last, I reached the no-bruise level. What is important is your response at the moment of your *duifang's* stinging hit. At

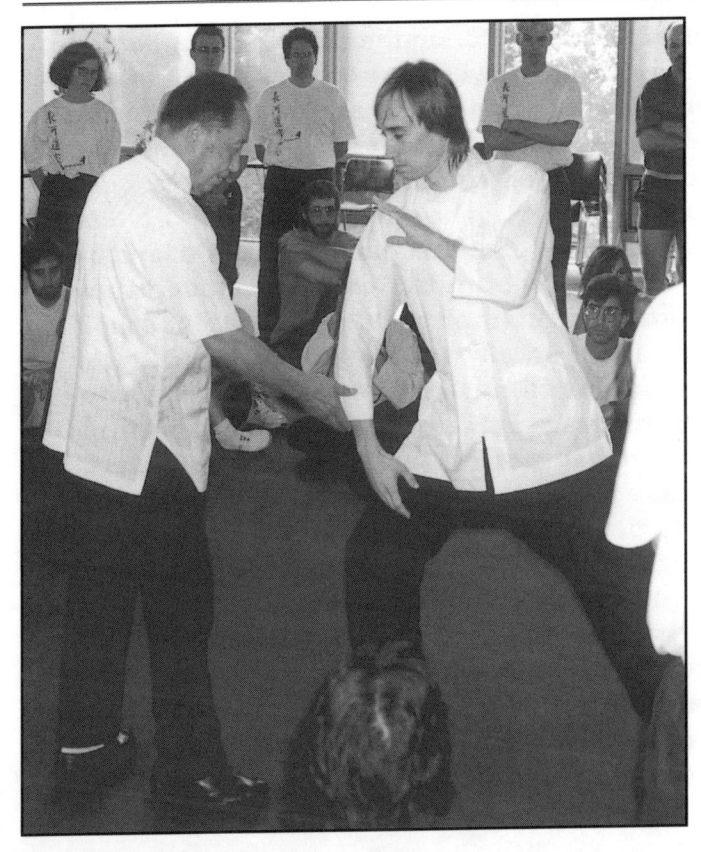

Wang Yen-nien explaining the proper body mechanics of *kao* (shoulder strike) with the author.

the beginning, anger, frustration, fear, pain, shame, and other emotions are sure to arise. They were there under the surface all the time. Now that they are in front of you, in the open, so is the opportunity to let go of them. It is a simple choice: apply the letting go you learned from *zhan zhuan* (standing post) and *tuishou,* or shrink back into the useless emotions that inhibit free movement.

For those practicing the martial way, I can think of no more useful practice than *sanshou* to polish and refine oneself for everyday life. Daily, we are assaulted by minor irritations, verbal attacks, and physical and emotional stress in all shapes and sizes. Most of these are not going to be as fast or furious as a potential palm in the face from a seasoned *taijiquan* player, but they might be as upsetting.

Once we lose our balance, it is usually not long before we act out of anger or some other emotion in a manner we regret and feel stupid about later. Having worked to achieve a calm mind amidst an onslaught of strikes, everyday problems are much easier to handle. Learning not to follow thought when stung in *sanshou*, it is easier to let go in the everyday. Learning to calmly deal with physical force coming at you through yielding and neutralizing makes learning to deal with more subtle forces a lot easier. Clearly, the physical is out in the open, the attack is obvious. Once you have learned to roll off a full-power punch to the nose without effort, or great amounts of muscle tension, or a change in your demeanor, then it is not such a big step to roll off all the other turmoil that life can rain down.

Let's face it, *fangsong*, letting go, softening, is a major goal of our *taijiquan* practice. It is easy to *fang song* on a spring day, strolling through the park with the flowers in bloom. I do not feel a great need for *taijiquan* then. It is the days when all hell breaks lose that we need our training. It is on those days that I thank Yang Luchan for passing on his art and *sanshou* practice for helping me to make the art real.

Conflict

The usual approach to martial arts is as a form of fighting - conflict - involving two forces colliding. We bring to our training all sorts of emotions. We concern ourselves with self-defense, defending the self, our ego. Conflict is the way we look at *sanshou* or any training that involves the martial application of our art. Yet it's all just motion, movement, momentum, and simply learning to let go of the self and change with that motion. It's learning to "see" the pattern of the movement and redirect it without forethought.

To move freely without inhibition, without thoughts in our way, requires us to flow with the motion of two people in action. Flow requires us to move with the pattern of events. In this, there is never really a self. Self is only our point of view. Self separates us, fools us into believing we are separate from all that is around us, especially the *duifang* before us. But we are just in the midst of the flow all the time, just like everything else. To work on martial arts only as self-defense is to lose the Way

Wang Yen-nien explaining the martial application of the Beat the Tiger movement with the author at the International *Taijiquan* Teachers' Workshop on the Applications of the *Yangjia Michuan* Style, Yuchih, Taiwan, 1991.

and develop only the small.

We must use *sanshou* to push past thought, past the self, into the stream of movement. In actuality, we are opening our eyes to where we always were. There, our *gongfu** flows. *Dao* is in harmony with the flow of events.

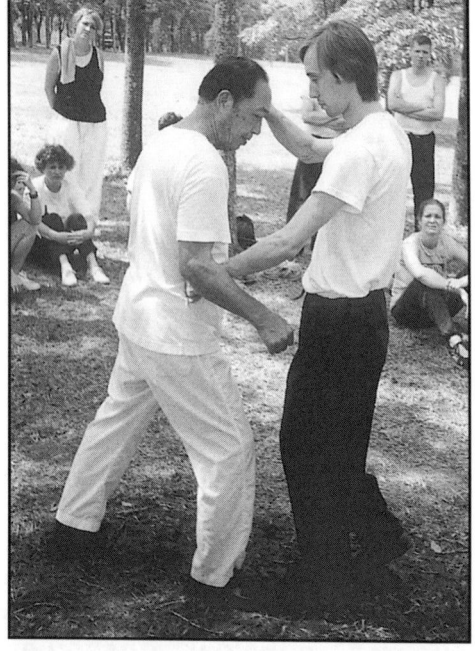

This is what makes our *gongfu* so grand. Not defending ourselves but losing the self completely, entering *wuwei* and following Laozi's example: "the sage does nothing but accomplishes everything." The sage seems to do nothing because he simply slides along the grain, follows the easy path, and rides it where he wants to go. And he does it without thinking about himself.

Sanshou - free hands - is our way to leap beyond.

* *Gongfu* is a Mandarin term, meaning "skill attained through long training."

Good and Bad Techniques

I remember a time when I was training at the first International *Taijiquan* Teachers' Workshop in Taiwan (1991). The workshop taught by Wang Yen-nien focused on the martial applications of the *Yangjia Michuan Taijiquan* system. I was working with a senior classmate on the uses of the Cloud Hands movement. Things were beginning to fall into place as we coached each other with feedback, noting when the attack was most controlled, etc.

Suddenly, we were approached by two other classmates who were not able to work the techniques. The older student watched for a while, analyzed our movements, and asked questions. After asking a few more questions, the senior student announced, "This doesn't work." I had overheard him saying this throughout the workshop, so after his pronouncement, I offered "Why not try it a few times and see what happens?" He screeched in all seriousness, "We've just been doing it for five minutes," and walked off. My partner and I looked at each other and burst out laughing.

There is no such thing as a correct technique that does not work. Certainly, there are movements that are more effective than others in certain situations, but movements would not have been preserved within traditional forms for hundreds of years if they were dead wood. Martial artists of the past could not afford the luxury of keeping movements because they were merely beautiful.

My classmate had missed the point. It is not whether a technique is "good" or not; it is whether our skill is at a level where we understand it enough, first structurally and, then, intuitively, to apply it. When a technique does not work, it is not like a pistol that has misfired. The problem is not with some external object. It is within ourselves. Cloud Hands is an extremely effective technique. My classmate failed because he sought the fault outside himself.

The same is true of martial arts in general. There is no such thing as the most effective martial art. Martial contests, and all other contests for that matter, depend most on the skill of the players. Just think about it. Judo, for example, is an excellent throwing art. But Judo can be neutralized by simply not letting the Judoko grab you. It's really that simple. But does that mean that a second or third year *taijiquan* student can defeat a third *dan* Jodoko with years of experience? Obviously not. He or she will be quickly thrown and, if lucky, not hurt.

The Cloud Hands episode reminds me of another time when I was practicing *Sanshou* at William C.C. Chen's school in New York City. I

Good and Bad...

was still a beginner then and playing against a more seasoned student. He threw a straight punch to my stomach. I instinctively turned my waist, deflecting with my forearm, and turned back, counter-striking with a backhand that found its target square on my partner's nose. He immediately stopped everything and gave me a ten-minute lecture on how a backhand punch is ineffective. I just listened quietly, smiling to myself.

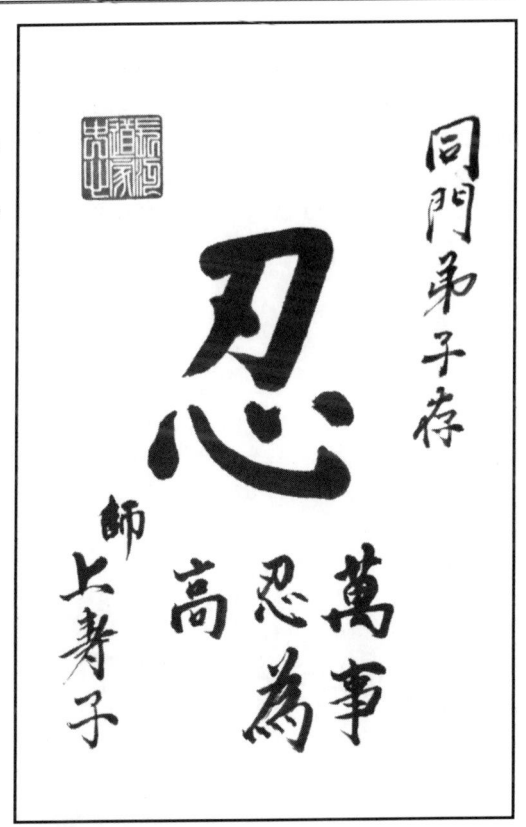

"Perseverance.
In ten thousand things, perseverance reaches the highest level"
signed Shang Shou Zi (Wang Yennien's Daoist name).

56

Understanding Li

Technique

The form's techniques must be practiced exactly. They have been preserved for centuries because they embody specific principles. But correct execution of technique is not the ultimate goal. Techniques are the vocabulary of our art. They are the way by which the principles are passed on. Deepening an understanding of technique is to deepen an understanding of principle. The point, however, is not merely a physically flawless performance of the form as if it is some sort of dance. Nor is it simply the conscious, meticulous practice of the form. The goal is an "unconscious," spontaneous application of the form/techniques in *tuishou* or *sanshou*. At this level, the techniques are not external, separate things to be performed. No dualism exists. We are the techniques, and the techniques are us, just as there is no feeling of separation of oneself and the *duifang*.*

What is the meaning of the principles underlying and creating *taijiquan*? Once, a student of mine, who also practiced *aikido*, was

*see *Tuishou* essay, page 41.

eager to show me a film of Ueshiba (the founder of *aikido*) practicing his solo spear techniques. As the film ran, the student commented on how Ueshiba had intensely studied the spear. Ueshiba felt that the movements he demonstrated represented "spiritual truths." That surprised me. For days I thought, "How can techniques for deflecting a spear and countering to kill another man embody spiritual truth?" Can techniques developed over centuries for the most effective method of killing contain spiritual insight? I felt compelled to answer this question and not simply toss it aside as the nonsensical observations of a junior student. It became my *koan*.*

Where do the principles of *taijiquan* lead us? Those who know our art completely understand how each deflection contains a counterstrike aimed at a point on the *duifang* that will do the most damage possible. To what kind of understanding do listening, joining, sticking, following, and releasing energy lead? Melding the techniques of form with the understanding of *tuishou*, one is led to an intuitive understanding of the pattern or grain of the body's movement. We train to develop continuous mind, an omnipresent awareness, while engaged in any activity. It is a physical, dynamic understanding of what the Chinese call *li*. The Mandarin term *li* is the natural pattern of things, such as the grain in wood or striations in jade. Through *taijiquan*, we reach toward an understanding of *li* not only in the human body but also in terms of dynamic forces in "conflict."

Techniques are a manifestation of *li* - the

---

*A paradox to be meditated upon.

Technique

underlying principles or pattern of the universe. Forcing things with muscle or brute force, working against the grain, is tiresome. Working against the grain reflects a lack of understanding of *li*. To deepen our technique is to deepen understanding.

When Laozi wrote of the sage undertaking no large tasks, dealing with no great problems, it sounds like the sage is a lazy bum who hides. On the contrary, the sage never works hard because he or she intuits the *li* or pattern of everyday life. Problems that appear as ripples in the pattern are dealt with while they are still ripples before they become tidal waves.

We *taijiquan* players must absorb principles and apply them to all spheres of life. What is practiced inside the *daochang* ("way hall," the Mandarin for practice hall) should be carried out the door and down the street, everywhere the player goes. Robert Smith told me once, "Whatever is outside in the world -- sunny days, thunder storms -- is also inside us. *Taijiquan* helps moderate the inside."

From a Daoist understanding of the universe, we know that everything is part of the Dao, the seamless web. Understanding the *li* of any art is understanding the pattern of the Dao in that context. The principles guiding our art lead to an understanding of our *li*, and from there lead to an understanding of the universal pattern that all things follow.

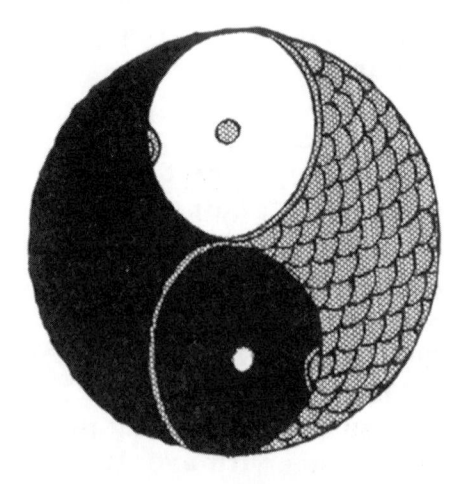

The Yang family *taiji* diagram.

Supermen and Common People

In his book, *Moving Zen: Karate as a Way to Gentleness*, Clive W. Nicol asked his teacher if he thought karate was the best unarmed combat. His teacher answered it was. Nicol had recently observed a *taijiquan* master named Wong easily toss Donn Draeger and other expert Budoka several feet across the room with "a simple-looking one-handed push that looked as harmless as the waking movements of a child." So he countered, "What about *taijiquan*?" Nakayama Sensei laughed, and with a smile, he said, "For human beings, Karate is the best way. But there are some men who are superhuman, and perhaps a few of the *Taiji* sensei are just that."

Taijiquan is so potentially transforming and evolutionary that masters of the art can appear quite superhuman. Attempting to push or punch them is like trying to beat up a cloud. And when they push back, releasing power, it's like a thunderbolt. Even with age, they not only do not run down, they get better. The last time I played *tuishou* with Wang Yen-nien, he was 84 (I was about a third his age). He said, "Come on, let me see how soft you are," and lined me up with my back to the wall. There was no one else around, so I was intent on testing myself and him. I knew I could not cause him any loss of face should I push him since we were alone. So I held nothing back and really tried to get him. Not only could I still not catch him, Wang pushed me into the wall three times and right down once. All the while, he let me try anything I liked to push him.

To put this in perspective, before I retired from competition, I won second place in international competition in *tuishou*. How many sports or other physical activities are there where a former, top-ranked player can be easily bested by a man three times his age?

When I asked Willam C.C. Chen what was the most important thing he learned from Cheng Man-ch'ing, he said, "Some people believe Cheng Man-ch'ing had super powers. But then when you lived with him (as Chen did), you discovered he was just a regular person. He was good, but he had some quality or method that made him that way." Of masters, Chen said, "They have two hands, and I have two hands." Chen credited these insights with his becoming a master. Before that, he thought he could never do it because Cheng appeared superhuman and he knew he (Chen) was not.

I have always aimed at mastery in my study of *taijiquan*. Chen's words not only encourage; they approve of mastery as a goal. Placing a teacher in the superhuman realm is tantamount to giving up. <u>We average humans</u>

Supermen and...

<u>know we are not genies with magic</u>. Placing the teacher high up in some god-like realm provides students a convenient excuse for not succeeding, for not even trying. For if we are just mortals, than we cannot be expected to perform like gods. Many times, I have heard a classmate describe some terrific skill he or she saw the teacher demonstrate, only to hear another say, "Well, that's Master Wang" -- as if somehow he has these skills because of *who* he is and not *how* he has practiced. The truth is that every master was born just as everyone else. In Wang's case, he practiced martial arts to strengthen himself because he was a sickly child. If anything, he started not with special gifts but with fewer gifts than the average child.

During a discussion of our goals in the martial arts with a fellow student, Paul Gallagher, I said, "I'm an arrogant student. I plan to reach my teacher's level and pass him." Paul replied, "You're not arrogant. There is no greater way for you to honor your teacher."

Alert, Inside and Out

"The form is that of a falcon about to seize a rabbit, and the *shen* is like that of a cat about to catch a rat."
-Wu Yu-xiang
Expositions of Insight into the Practice of the Thirteen Postures

How can you concentrate on the inside, on the *dantian*, and, at the same time, be watching the outside, aware of what is going on around you?

When practicing the form or push hands, we must constantly be alert and mindful of the *duifang* and our surroundings. Yang Luchan said, "Always heed." At the same time, when practicing the form, the mind must reside in the *dantian*, activating its pump-like qualities to circulate the *qi* throughout the body. This apparent conflict of focus, inside and out, is resolved in two ways.

The first way is that though the eyes are watching and seeing everything, they are not focusing on anything. The eyes do not go out to any object or movement. The eyes do not develop any attachments. The eyes are joined to the surroundings like blotters. Everything travels into the eyes and other senses equally. All vision is as peripheral vision. Not focusing on one thing, not going out to it, the senses take in everything. Secondly, since the eyes are not going out, the intent is not going out, therefore, all the while, the mind perches on and resides in the *dantian*.

Training to reach this level is like learning any other skill or developing the body in any other way. When we first learn to ride a bike, it seems an impossible task that requires all our attention. After a week of riding, anyone can zoom along, weaving in and out of obstacles, and concentrating on anything he or she chooses.

When the method of concentrating the mind in the *dantian* has been trained and developed so that it is completely natural, the mind can also be entirely focused on watching the *duifang* or being aware of and "joined" with the surroundings when there is no *duifang*.

As with other skills developed through practice, holding to the *dantian* and being continuously aware is layered upon and into skills that have been integrated into the body/mind.

Mistakes

"Timidness is not correct,
Bravery is not correct,
Strong Courage and Keen Perception are
Correct."
Song of Perfect Clarity
-*Yang Family Transmissions*
Douglas Wile, trans.

    Take the opportunity to make mistakes during practice. Have the daring to stand in front of the class with the teacher's eyes on you. This is your chance to test and refine what you know before the ultimate test of competition on the street.

    Always standing in the back, never volunteering to demonstrate for the class or to lead, robs the student of his or her most valuable training tool - the critical eye of the teacher and classmates. Anyone can be relaxed and calm practicing in a field of flowers. Who needs *taijiquan* then? Life is full of flowers, but we all know this is only a part of life. At times, it is only a small part. We need our art for the thunderstorms more than the sunny days. The daring to place ourselves in a position where we will be criticized, to open ourselves up under pressure, is a genuine opportunity to discover our weaknesses.

Willingness to make mistakes in the supportive environment of your own center, *dojo,* or *daochang* is a good first challenge for the martial artist or any type of artist. Past warriors were tested with steel; they never or rarely fought the same adversary twice. In modern competition, one's opponent rarely offers aid (gives you what you need to face him or her the next time). The practice hall is one of the very few environments where one gets a second or even a third chance or the help of the *duifang*.

Injury

Once in applications class, I had the good luck to practice with a classmate who had a great deal of fighting experience -- a champion. The unfortunate price I paid was that while practicing leg sweeps, my calf was hurt. After dinner, it began to stiffen up and ache. Walking to *tuishou* class, I was running the age-old debate every dedicated practitioner has had in my mind. Am I too hurt to practice? Will I make it worse by playing? Am I just giving myself an excuse to be lazy?

Sometimes, it is hard to give yourself a rest, to wait. So I decided to sit it out and not take any chances. While I was sitting watching the explanation of tournament rules for fixed-step push hands, I was also working on my Chinese so I'd know what to say if my teacher called my name. The next player called up was Christian, an excellent player. I thought Robert, another classmate, would be a great match for him (they are both bigger than I am). All of a sudden, the teacher called my name. I stood up, shook out, drew in *qi* to my *dantian,* and leaped into the ring. I was exhilarated and ready to play.

It is this spirit that is a dividing line among martial artists. There are those of us who cannot wait to probe, test, and challenge ourselves. Our spirit pulls us forward. Sometimes, we are pulled into play when we should sit, and we pay for it with injuries. While we admonish ourselves for not being more sensitive to our bodies or, more precisely, not paying attention to the senses we have developed, we know it is this same drive that carries us up, the same spirit that raises our *gongfu*. And we are afraid of losing it.

Maybe when we are masters we will rest and wait. Maybe that is how we will know we are masters.

Tournament Competition

Every criticism of *taiji* tournaments is correct. These criticisms typically revolve around the observation that most competitors replaced aggression and muscle strength for anything that might resemble *taijiquan*. The worst part of the push hands competition is that often the winner has displayed not even a single technique of *taijiquan* and displayed even fewer *taiji* principles, such as yielding and neutralizing. Matches tend to look more like sumo than *taijiquan*. And worst of all, these "champions" are approached as experts in the art.

Yet I have been active in tournaments from the local to international level. Furthermore, I have required intermediate students to play in at least one tournament a year. Our *taijiquan* school has sponsored a yearly competition. Students are also encouraged to play *tuishou* and *sanshou* at other schools.

How can I be in complete agreement with every criticism of tournaments and yet require my students to play in them? It's a matter of approach. Most players, perhaps 99 percent, enter tournaments to win. They enter to make their names prior to opening up schools. Entering the ring, they lose their minds. Yielding is forgotten, and shoving becomes the rule. So much seems to be at stake. There is not a relaxed person in the gymnasium.

When I entered the ring or when I send in a student, it is a test, a challenge. What is important is the play, not securing victory.

Anyone can be relaxed outside on a beautiful day, walking through the park picking flowers. We don't need our *taijiquan* on those days. Unfortunately, most days aren't spent amongst the flowers. People are constantly trying to push us over one way or another - verbally, physically and emotionally.

Stepping into the tournament ring means knowingly facing a *duifang* who is just that, not a friendly training partner. Each player is going to face naked aggression from someone who is going to seem absolutely lunatic. And it might not be just the other player in that ring; it may be ourselves who go mad. And though push hands is supposed to be a friendly game, in competition, injury is common. Now the question is, faced with an unfriendly match in unfamiliar surroundings, are you going to lose it and face stiff, muscular aggression with more of the same? Fire against fire? Has this been your training in *taijiquan*? Will you apply your training or forget it under stress?

The challenge is to do *taijiquan*. The challenge is to be *taijiquan*. When you are pushed

Tournament Competition

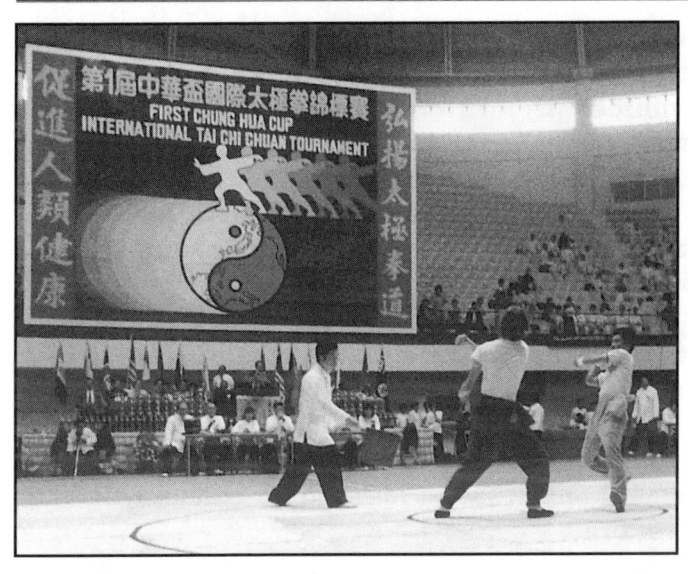

The author, on left, competing at the First Cheng Hua International Tournament in 1990.

or knocked to the ground, does your ego rise and body stiffen? Do you rush forward without listening? And if you violate everything you have espoused as a student, if every one of your teacher's lessons took flight during the match, what will you do afterward? Tournaments are a true test and an excellent learning experience -- that is, if we choose to listen to the experience. I cannot count the number of times I have heard complaints after the match: "He just used force"; "He didn't use *taijiquan*." Everyone is walking around complaining that his or her good *taijiquan* lost to someone's bad *taijiquan*. Are these players listening to themselves? Are they saying that their art only works when the attacker plays by their rules or only works on sunny days in the park?

I laugh when someone attacks me like a freight train. Most students fear this kind of attack. It's just more energy with which to throw them. If we study every day that yielding and softness neutralizes the stiff and hard, then complain when we are unable to apply our beautiful philosophy, which has failed - ourselves or our art?

After a tournament, win or lose, sit down quietly, send your ego out for a walk, and ask: Did I relax? Was I soft in the face of aggression? Did I follow my own philosophy and training or revert to anger, giving into aggression and stiffness? Answering yes or no, are you still probing for how to deepen your practice? Will you strive to really answer your own aggression and stiffness? Will any lessons learned be lost during the next match?

Self-mastery will take daring; it requires investing in loss. Or as the *Song of Perfect Clarity* explains, "Timidity is not correct, Bravery is not correct, strong courage and keen perception are correct."

A match is a cold bucket of water dumped over your head. Do you choose to wake up? There are no greater tests or measures of *taiji gongfu* anywhere outside of a real life-and-death struggle on the street. The choice is to face this challenge and honestly evaluate our *gongfu* or not to. Is pointing fingers and accusing others of debasing our art a method of self-cultivation? Is *taijiquan* practiced for self-mastery or to prove who is most philosophically correct? The question is not whether having tournaments is correct or incorrect but how to make use of tournaments for our individual progress in this art.

Fear

What is fear? Every martial artist has to face it. Every martial artist must overcome it. To overcome fear, we must know what fear is.

Fear is losing being present. Fear is projecting into the future. Why is it that ordinary people can undertake heroic acts? "There wasn't time to think," they say. People leap into situations and do what they thought was impossible without thinking. If anyone had thought about it, not a single person would have run into a building ablaze to save a child. And if one did run into a burning building while contemplating one's chances, he would not have the awareness needed to save himself or anyone else.

Thinking drowns us in a world of "what ifs;" it pulls us into imagined futures -- futures that don't exist. Only the present moment exists. Losing the present, giving way to fear, we lose our capabilities because we are not here.

Fear kills mindfulness.

Opponents

As martial artists, we strive for total mastery of our art. Reaching absolute mastery of outward skill is our means of self-mastery. To be a master of our art or any art is to be a master of one's self, of the self.

Along our journey, we face many opponents for many reasons. We even face obstacles when it is not necessary. But there is no greater opponent we face than ourselves. No individual, no group can truly put any obstacle in our path. The teacher lives too far away -- move. No one to practice with -- teach someone up to your level. No time -- throw the television out the window. Tired from work and family -- practice to strengthen body and mind. No one supports your practice, and they believe you're crazy -- toss out attachment.

There are no problems or reasons why anyone cannot practice and succeed if he or she is willing to face his or her strongest opponent.

In all my matches, I have faced no greater

opponent than myself. I am my only real opponent.

Selected Readings

...On *taijiquan*:

Lo, Benjamin P. J. and Inn, Martin, trans., *Cheng Tzu's Thirteen Treatises on T'ai Chi Ch'uan*, Berkeley: North Atlantic Book, 1985. isbn: 0938190458.

Liang, T. T., *T'ai Chi Ch'uan For Health and Self-Defense, Philosophy and Practice*, New York: Vintage Books, 1977, isbn: 0394724615. *An excellent, plain language version of the classics along with Master Liang's commentary and important ideas in taijiquan.*

Lo, Benjamin P. J. and Smith, Robert W. trans., *T'ai Chi Ch'uan Ta Wen, Questions and Answers on T'ai Chi Ch'uan*, Berkeley: North Atlantic Books, 1985. isbn: 0938190679.

Davis, Barbara, *The Taijiquan Classics: An Annotated Translation*, Berkeley, North Atlantic Books: 2004. isbn: 1556434316.

Lowenthal, Wolfe, *There Are No Secrets*,

Professor Cheng Man-ch'ing and his T'ai Chi Chuan, Berkeley: North Atlantic Books, 1991. isbn: 1556431120. *A wonderful introspective view on personal development in taijiquan and Cheng Man-ch'ing.*

Lowenthal, Wolfe, *Gateway to the Miraculous: Further Explorations in the Tao of Cheng Man-Ch'ing.* Frog Ltd., 1994. isbn: 1883319137.

Olson, Stuart A., trans., *The Wind Sweeps Away the Plum Blossoms, Principles and Techniques of the Yang Style T'ai Chi Spear and Staff*, Winnipeg: Bubbling Well Press, 1985. isbn: 0938045008.

Rodell, Scott M., *Chinese Swordsmanship· The Yang Family Taiji Jian Tradition*, Annandale: Seven Stars Books and Video, 2003. isbn: 0-9743999-0-6.

Wang, Yen-nien, *Yangjia Michuan Taijiquan Tujie, Shiyongfa* (Yang Family Secret Transmission Taiji Fist, Martial Applications), Taipei, 1996, isbn: 957-99475-1-1.

Wile, Douglas, trans., *T'ai-Chi Touchstones: Yang Family Secret Transmissions*, Brooklyn: Sweet Ch'i Press, 1983. isbn: 091205901X. *The only English translation of important Yang family treatises.*

...On the Martial Path:

Almeida, Bira, *Capoeira, A Brazilian Art Form*, Berkeley: North Atlantic Books, 1986. isbn: 0938190296.

Selected Readings

Evangelista, Nick, *The Inner Game of Fencing, Excellence in Form, Technique, Strategy and Spirit*, Chicago: Masters Press, 2000, isbn 1-57028-230-7.

Fields, Rick, *The Code of the Warrior, In Myth, And Everyday Life*. Harper Collins Publishers, 1991, isbn: 006096605X.

Nicol, Clive W., *Moving Zen - Karate as a Way to Gentleness*, London: The Body Head Ltd., 1975. isbn: 0688011810. *Ever wonder what its like to travel to another country and train with all you got? Read this book.*

Stevens, John, *The Sword of No Sword*, Boulder: Shambhala, 1984, isbn: 1570620504. *Depicts the life of a warrior completely dedicated to enlightenment.*

Heckler, Richard S., *In Search of the Warrior Spirit*, Berkeley: North Atlantic Books, 1990. isbn: 1556434251. *Probing and questioning debate on the role of the warrior in modern society and in the military.*

Mark V. Wiley, *Filipino Martial Culture*, Singapore: Charles E. Tuttle Publishing, 1997. isbn: 0804820880. *An excellent study of the Filipino tradition that sets a standard for other arts.*

Scott M. Rodell is the Director of the Great River Taoist Center, which he founded in '84. Great River (http://www.grtc.org/) is headquartered in Washington, D.C., and has branches in the US and across Northern Europe.

He began teaching in the Soviet Union at the request of the Soviet *Wushu* Federation in '91. In '92, the Moscow school officially opened as a branch of Great River with groups later forming in other Russian and Estonian cities.

He was also one of the first ten Americans to enter the door of the *Jin Shan Pai*, a traditional school of Daoist *neigong*. Rodell, initiated into the *Jin Shan Pai* by Wang Yen-nien, is a sixth-generation teacher in this tradition.

Some highlights of Rodell's career include:
° Began studying martial arts at nine years of age. Rodell practiced Karate, Judo, Tournament & Instinct Archery, Wrestling, Sport Fencing, & Marksmanship before devoting his training full-time to *taijiquan*.
° Has over 20 years of *taijiquan* training in two branches of Yang *Taijiquan*.
° Studied with several senior students of Zheng Manqing, including noted masters William C.C. Chen & T.T. Liang. He studied push hands & free fighting with Chen & push hands & sword with Liang. Rodell is also a disciple student of Master Wang Yen-nien of Shanxi province with whom he studied all aspects of Yang family *Michuan* (Secret Teaching) Taijiquan.
° During the late '80s, he was Push Hands Champion at several nationally sanctioned tournaments & placed second in Push Hands at the International Championship held in the Republic of China in '91.
° Has been teaching regular seminars from beginners *taijiquan* to advanced Chinese Swordsmanship in Europe since '91.
° Awarded "Honored Judge" rank by the Russian Wushu Federation (their highest rank), 2001.
° Proprietor of Seven Stars Trading Co. (http://www.sevenstarstrading.com/), specializing in Imperial Chinese arms & armor.
° Moderator, Chinese Swords & Swordsmanship Forum, *Sword Forum International* (SwordForum.com).